My Son
A Gift from God

My Son
A Gift from God

❖

Jack Pusch

Library of Congress Control Number:		2010905578
ISBN:	Hardcover	978-1-4500-8725-4
	Softcover	978-1-4500-8724-7
	Ebook	978-1-4500-8726-1

To order additional copies of this book, contact:
Xlibris Corporation
1-888-795-4274
www.Xlibris.com
Orders@Xlibris.com
75418

CONTENTS

Preface 9

Chapter 1   My Preteen Years 11

Chapter 2   Teenage to Manhood 15

Chapter 3   My Military Life 16

Chapter 4   My Father 26

Chapter 5   My Mother 28

Chapter 6   My Return to Civilian Life 29

Chapter 7   Bill, the Lawyer 38

Chapter 8   Bill, the Businessman 40

Chapter 9   Bill in Banking 43

Chapter 10   Bill the Person 49

Chapter 11   Conclusion 51

Epilogue 57

Index 59

About the Cover

"Bill peeling potatoes for his Dad on Thanksgiving Day, 2004, shortly before his death."

A reminder for us all.

Jim Osborne, a deacon in my church came to see me about a week after Bill died. I was about as down as a man can get. Jim brought up the relative lack of importance of our collectables in life, compared to having Bill still alive and here with me.

I will always be very grateful to him for that visit, a very meaningful occasion in my life.

PREFACE

This book is dedicated to God, our Father in Heaven, whom we never give enough credit. He is always there to comfort us and see us through the best and the worst happenings in life; to my father Edwin Kurt Pusch, a good and decent man who overcame many obstacles and always did the right thing, even as he was being taken advantage of by the Andersons who used him and cursed him for many years; and my son William L. Pusch who never let health or any adverse happenings stand in his way and went on to be a model Son, husband, father, business man, lawyer and Christian.

Bill wanted me to write a book about myself as he thought I'd been told I was such a dummy, yet I had given him good advice. He thought I'd survived my rough childhood well and had good judgment and make good decisions.

I'm sure I never would have written a book about me but since I was writing about him I want to let people know to never to give up. To anyone who reads this just remember, you are a failure in life only if you allow yourself to be. To succeed you only have to do what is right and do the best you can, God isn't impressed by our wealth, only our character.

My lack of education kept me from making a better salary but my goal was to always to do what is right and I sleep well.

The one thing I want to convey is what a consistent regard my Bill had for others.

I have always been concerned about fairness when dealing with others. I noticed when Bill was very young that he always had that concern about how things affected other people. He thought I was hardnosed and I would tell him that I shared his concern for others but in the course of life we do have to get serious and do the things that need to be done. As he grew into maturity I could see he was grasping the realities of life and finally recognized that some people are never going to be responsible. For all, but especially the young who may read this I want them to grasp this reality.

The real point I wish to convey though is that my Bill, having experienced The disappointments of life like having to give up flying because of Diabetes never gave up, never said, why me, or felt he deserved special consideration because of his disappointments in life.

CHAPTER 1

My Preteen Years

My mother, Allene Pusch, died at Picher, Oklahoma, on May 22, 1935, during a surgical procedure. After her death, my brother and I went to live with my maternal grandparents, L. D. and Lula Bell Anderson, in Russellville, Arkansas. We lived in the poorest part of town, known as Hell's Half Acre. My brother Arthur was about a year older than I was; I was about twenty months old at the time.

I think it was about 1937 or 1938, that my father bought eighty acres of land on Shinn Mountain, about five miles west of Dover, and moved us and the Andersons there. I think my dad's thinking was it would be a good idea to get my grandfather removed from easy access to booze and the fact that in the country he could have a garden to grow some of our food.

The old shack we lived in had no running water or electricity. A two-holer outside served as our toilet. We used Montgomery Ward and Sears catalogs as toilet paper. We had a spring that was our source of water. It had a terra-cotta tile about three feet in diameter and three feet deep down in the ground that had a chip on one side to allow the excess water to flow out. We had a two-gallon water bucket that we dipped into the well to obtain our household water. We all drank from the bucket via a dipper that everyone used. Primitive it was, but as I told my Bill later, we did what we had to. The spring was known about by lots of people, and people would stop by from time to time to see the spring again.

My brother's first four years and my first three years, we walked about a mile and a half to a one-room school located out in the woods where it was centered to accommodate kids surrounding it. Beginning in my fourth grade, we began riding a bus to the grammar school in Dover.

Our clothing like everything else was about as cheap as we could find. I always wanted Levi's jeans, but they cost too much; we had something from Sears, Montgomery Ward, or hand-me-downs. How I was ever elected to class officer positions in the Dover school system still amazes me.

The Andersons were bitter old people who had once been wealthy enough to have servants; someone who drove the kids to school in a buggy, I was told by my uncle Burford; and in general were enjoying the life of very successful businesspeople. Being with them, we could always count on someone being cussed. They seemed to hate everyone who had done well in life. As I grew older and heard family names, if they were successful and well-known, many times they had been repeatedly cussed by Grandfather.

They were so bitter from the first I knew of them; even though my father provided them a place to live and money to live on, they cussed my father all the time. My grandfather was the meanest old man I have ever seen. He was so cruel that when he fed his hogs, who were half-starved, he would use a stick with a razor blade attached to the end of it to cut the hogs' noses as they came scrambling for food.

My grandmother told me that in the good times when they had money, my grandfather would go uptown each night carrying two pistols. Supposedly he had killed a man once. I don't swear anymore, but I still describe him as the meanest old SOB I have ever seen.

After I grew up, I could understand part of the Andersons' anger. They had been on top, and then they were dependent on my dad for their very existence. Their children provided very little financial assistance to them. They were content to let my dad carry the financial load that had been imposed upon him.

What was telling about the Anderson boys was that except for the youngest, Elmer, who was not very intelligent, was the only one to really try to help them. At least he had the decency to try to assist them.

My grandfather was an alcoholic, and my grandmother loved to drink also. I am sure that a lot of the money provided by my father for us all to live on was spent on booze. They drank every chance they got. I would defend my father when he was cussed, and they in turn got their revenge by telling me how stupid I was and how intelligent my brother was. I'm glad in hindsight that I stood up to them as I later learned what a wonderful man my father was.

Two baby boys living with the Andersons was a terrible place for young kids to be in. Unfortunately, they still drank a lot when they had the money, and when one of their kids came home, we could count on a terrible drunken fight.

Since I stood up to them when they cussed my dad, I was an easy target for their anger. So the whippings I got, which I later figured out to be them taking their hatred for Dad out on me never let up. Most telling was when my brother, who was a year older than me, had a fight and I lost, I got a whipping and was told I would in the future until I whipped him.

You couldn't call their treatment of me brutal; it wasn't that bad, but a child shouldn't have to live that way. Though Bill was upset when he heard about it, and I sure didn't like it, I really think it helped make me a stronger man, gave a feeling for others, and I'm sure made me take my duties more seriously in life. I was determined to do whatever I was assigned to do and to do it well. I think it played a role in me being recognized by top management people as being one whose ideas mattered, and I could always be counted on to get the job done.

At that time, neither they nor I knew that my Bill would later come into my life and bring a joy that all the prior misery could never erase.

After I grew up, I decided I was not going to be anyone's punching bag. I let it be known that if someone was going to get the best of me, it would be after a battle. For those who encounter what I did, just remember, you have a choice; you can let those who would harm you do it, or as I did, take what you have to, but never let them break your will to live an independent life and seek happiness.

Other than my mother, the Andersons had one daughter (Louise) and sons (William, Vernon, Burford, and Elmer). Other than my mother, all their kids were messed up somehow; most of them drank and in general were no good. My uncle Burford was so tight that I think he worshipped the penny, not the dollar. His love of money was greater than that for his own family. He made no effort to attend his sister Louise's nor his brother Elmer's funeral. To me he had a heart of stone.

This all started during the Depression, and my dad was really carrying a financial load since he had agreed to let the Andersons have us kids. In order to support us kids, he had to support them also. My dad would tell me later that he wanted to put my brother and me in a Catholic school for children, but the Andersons wanted us. As I got older, I figured out why; with us, my dad would support them also.

We were so poor that once, I was reminded by a newcomer kid to the area that I was wearing a girl's blouse. We were poor enough that we took hand-me-downs and wore what we could get.

My grandparents had lost their wealth and good social standing long before my father married my mother. I was later told that my mother was a wonderful, caring woman who was loved by lots of people because she was such a sweet person. My uncles, except Burford, and my aunt were mostly like their parents in that they also loved to drink. When any of them would come home, there was usually a drunken fight among all of them. What an environment to raise two young boys in!

During one of my grandfather's drunken states, he decided to go beat my father up with a blackjack. My dad was visiting and stayed in another shack on an adjoining forty-acre tract of land he had bought. I estimate I was under the age of ten by trying to review that time. My grandfather said he was going to do something to that GD flat-headed Dutchman. As he walked by me, I grabbed the blackjack out of his hand and took it out where my brother and I cut wood (to burn for cooking and heating) and cut the blackjack with an axe, and most of the lead pellets came out of it. Looking back and being young, I'm really proud that my next move was to take the remaining cut-up leather back and hand it to my grandfather. He was shocked that I stood up to him so dramatically, and I'll never forget the shocked look on his face. My brother asked me why I did what I did, which I didn't answer.

What I'm most proud of is that at that early age I could see and understand the load my father carried trying to provide a home for my brother and me, and the lack of appreciation the Andersons had for his providing them a living, meager it was; they had a place to live and food to eat. My grasp of the situation then, I think, laid the groundwork for my being able to help my dad make decisions when he had to quit work, and later financially. I just saw it as my duty to help him. I glad I did. This prepared me later to assess what was going on and manage places, successfully, that had not been run well.

My brother was the Andersons' favorite, and he played it safe and never offended them, but I took up for my father when my grandfather would cuss him. Needless to say, I was not in good standing, and they would call me a Pusch and my brother an Anderson.

Unfortunately they were correct in that he became an alcoholic also, and the booze killed him at the age of fifty-eight. What was sad about him was he had a good mind but was only interested in what he wanted and was never aggressive about getting ahead.

Anyway, it was a very difficult childhood, but somehow we survived it. I was determined that they would not ruin my life.

Chapter 2

Teenage to Manhood

My father's health failed when I was about fifteen years old, and I had to start helping provide for his welfare. The Andersons were gone by this time, and I was living out in the sticks alone. When my dad came there, we talked and decided that the only way he could get enough money to live on was for me to go into the army so I could, with the army's help, provide him sufficient extra money to live on. At that time, if I put up so much money, the army would supplement it through an allotment system for dependent parents. I was just a dumb country kid who had quit school in the tenth grade and knew nothing about the real world. Until my dad joined me, I had only heard how dumb I was from the Andersons but had been well received in school. I guess today I would be seen as needing counseling. I don't know my thinking, but I guess I believed I was really inferior to my peers even though I had been elected to several class officer positions over the years in school. I had quit school after being out with the flu before I completed the tenth grade.

The old shack we lived in was about to fall down, so we decided to tear it down, reuse most of the lumber, and build a smaller house for my father to live in. So we moved into another shack with a neighbor so I could tear the old shack down. I'm proud that as a fifteen- or sixteen-year-old I was mature enough to tear the old house down, and I built a rock foundation for the new house and then hired a carpenter who provided the skill for him and me to build the new house, a better shack.

Then my father decided that with some laying hens he could supplement his income by selling eggs, so I built him a chicken house also. By that time I was about seventeen and a half years old, and my father gave his permission for me to enter the U.S. Army on February 13, 1951.

CHAPTER 3
My Military Life

I was sent to Fort Chaffee, near Fort Smith, Arkansas, and attended the army's cook and bakers school at Fort Chaffee. In late 1952 I was transferred to Fort Sill at Lawton, Oklahoma. While stationed there, I married Retha Mae Winders on October 20, 1952. This was the beginning of a contentious thirty-three-year marriage.

I didn't think about it at the time, but as an army cook, I was surrounded by a bunch of drunks again, as I had been while being raised by the Andersons. I was only at Fort Sill a few months and was sent to Korea in January 1953. When I got there, I was assigned to the 45th Infantry Division's 120th Ambulance Company of the 120th Medical Battalion to work as cook.

After I got there, I discovered an alcoholic master sergeant was the mess sergeant and the next highest-ranking man was a corporal. At that time I was a PFC, a one-striper. Even though I was the lowest-ranking person there, I immediately began to learn from the sergeant how things got done. I started doing all the paperwork and taking it to the turn-in point at the end of each day. I guess since I had to help my dad, it was just natural to jump in and help get the job done.

A month or two after I got there, the sergeant got drunk and stayed that way for several days. In spite of me being the lowest-ranking person there, I took over his job, by basically continuing to do what I was already doing. My commander knew who was doing the work, so he officially put me in charge, with higher-ranking people working for me. They promoted me three times that year and gave me a Bronze Star for my duty performance.

People older than me found it hard to work for someone as young as I was. I had a first sergeant that was afraid I was going to be promoted higher in rank than he was, and he tried hard to make my life miserable and succeeded, to some extent, for a short period of time. We had a cook who was forty-two years old, and he really found it hard to take that I was in charge. I was nineteen at the time. One day he proceeded to tell me that he was old enough to be my father and was continuing when I cut him off. I informed him that I didn't promote him or myself and he could be sure I was going to do my job and he had better do his, and with that the conversation was over.

In that time, if we failed in a job, there were consequences, reductions in rank, or some action to punish our failure. Seventeen years later, just prior to my retirement from the air force, I had to go clean up a mess, and those who caused the problem weren't held accountable for their failure to get the job done. Our country is paying a price for this laxness. Personal responsibility is just as important today as it was then.

While in Korea we moved a couple of times, and when the war ended, I was moved into a metal building. It had a dirt floor, but at least we were out of a tent.

The 120th Medical Clearing Company a sister unit was a MASH-type unit that provided the first available surgical care about ten miles behind the front lines during the war. By this time, they were located close to us. They had all the division's surgeons, dentists, and related health-care providers. They had their own officers' mess hall, but most of the doctors liked my food better and always wanted to eat at my mess hall. I had limited rations and had transients going through to eat, so I could only feed a few extras. Most of the time I would tell them to only send me two or three at a time for the noon meal. They cooperated with me, and it worked out well.

I finally made arrangements with our quartermaster people to provide me with enough steak for all the officers and all my people about one every two or three months for an evening meal. Since I was known for producing good food, the steak was just the icing on the cake.

Of course, the menu showed that I had fed the recommended Army Master Menu meal. When I first took over the mess tent, I had fed better food than was recommended and was nearly court-martialed for it. I told the colonel at quartermaster about that, and I think he figured we could get by with doing it now that the war was over. I think the only thing that saved me from being court-martialed was that I had the won the Best Mess award for several months, presented by the commanding general. Many years later, I told my Bill about this and the fact that they probably finally figured out that they would look like fools punishing me after acknowledging I was doing such a good job.

On the several occasions that year when being awarded the plaque for having the best mess hall in the 45th Infantry Division by the commanding general, I was usually the first to report to him as he landed close to me. My company commander and battalion commander would come running to get there as soon as possible.

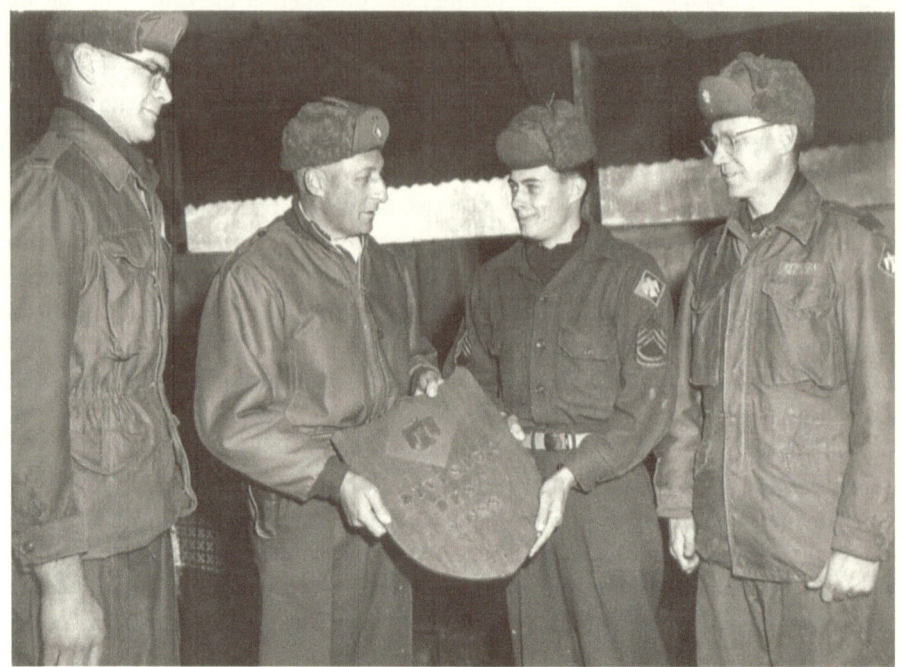

SFC Jack Pusch receiving Best Mess Award from Major General Paul Harkins,
Commanding General, 45th Infantry Division.

During one of those awards, Brigadier General J. F. R. Seitz, the only one-star division commander I had ever seen, offered to show me how to make mayonnaise. I think I had the oil but no vinegar, and we couldn't do it. Here he was, a division commander, one of the nicest people I had ever met in the army going to show this kid something. I never thought about it at the time, but I guess if the Andersons could have seen what was going on, they would have been shocked.

I am proud of the fact that my company commander in Korea wanted me to become an officer. He told me I needed to be "one of us," as he put it, and I asked him what he meant and he said "an officer." I told him I had not completed the tenth grade when I was married, and I think I said "screwed."

Later he thought he had it all figured out; Fort Rucker, in Alabama, wanted to train noncommissioned officers like me to become helicopter pilots. There was one hitch; I wasn't twenty and a half years old. He said, "You mean to tell me one of my senior NCOs is not that old?" I told him, "Yeah, that is the way it was." Soon after that, he told me he was leaving, but my next promotion was assured. Soon after that, I was promoted again to E-6, sergeant first class, one step under a master sergeant. That year in Korea assured me I was capable of performing well under adverse conditions.

When my time came to return to the USA, I had reached the age of twenty. My battalion commander came to me to tell me that if I would extend my tour in Korea two more months, he would promote me to the rank of master sergeant, the army's highest enlisted rank at that time. I told him I appreciated his offer, but I had a recently born son whom I had never seen and needed to go home, so I returned to the USA in January 1954.

During my time in Korea, my father would write me and tell me he couldn't keep up with my rank as it changed so often. I guess a good way to put it was he was as proud as I was surprised how many promotions I received that year.

Knowing that I didn't have an education to qualify me for something better, I decided that joining the air force was my best choice for a career. I did not want to supervise a bunch of drunken army cooks even though it was very likely that I would have been promoted to the warrant officer rank. They acted like they had never seen anyone as aggressive as me. The top-ranked warrant officer pay was about equal to a major's pay, but I would have still been involved with a bunch of drunken cooks.

My first assignment in the air force was to Barksdale Air Force Base, at Bossier City, Louisiana. I requested and was assigned to do personnel work. I was surprised how I was treated by the ranking noncommissioned officers, mostly master sergeants who had served in WWII. Even though I had to drop two pay grades, they treated me as if I were one of them. They were apparently impressed that I had achieved the rank I had in the army. They were more impressed when I was awarded the Bronze Star. Receiving the award was unpleasant as after the parade while awaiting the award I nearly passed out in the Louisiana sun.

Again it sunk in that I was more capable than I had been told when I was a child.

One of the saddest things in my life occurred on July 19, 1954, when my father, Edwin Kurt Pusch, died. I did not really get to know my father well until his health failed and I had to start helping him. When I was really young, he would come home dressed in a suit, which we saw little of, and would bring gifts, candy, nuts, fruit, and things we seldom saw. When we started living together, I learned what a good and decent man he really was. When he died, I grieved like never before because I had lost a friend and father. I had never had a friend in the family before. My wife was certainly never a friend. I never had one again until my Bill was born.

While stationed at Barksdale, my second son, Steven Kurt Pusch, was born on January 18, 1955. In August 1955, I was assigned to Homestead Air Force Base, at Homestead, Florida. This was quite a shock as I had never been to a tropical area, and prices were very high.

I was the sixteenth person to arrive at the base, and it was quite an experience establishing a new base.

While at Barksdale, I had been trained to evaluate and determine where people do their most effective work in the air force. I didn't have much personnel experience, but at Homestead I was the noncommissioned officer in charge of the classification and testing section of the base personnel shop. My boss, Jack Mathews, was a first lieutenant, formerly an enlisted man, who really didn't want to be an officer. He showed little interest in his job and often stated that he missed being one of the enlisted men and didn't want to associate with officers. I wanted to be an officer badly, but my commander just never could find a way to make it happen.

While at Homestead, I learned a lot about people. That was a very interesting and dangerous period of time for our country. Russia was taking over Eastern Europe, and in our particular case at Homestead, we were in the process of developing a large Strategic Air Command base, which when done would have two B-47 bomber wings and the support functions. Russia had developed a hydrogen bomb, and we were in a rush to build up a large bomber force to counteract anything that they did.

I had had to grow up young in order to help my dad, but there was a lot about life I had not experienced. At Homestead I would be working with a senior officer one day and the next he would be dead. There was so much pressure on us to get bomb squadrons combat ready that a lot of people were killed during test flights near the base. As in Korea where I saw a lot of injured and dead, it came to me more and more the price our military personnel pay to protect our way of life. Those privileged people who attend elitist schools should get an understanding of real life before criticizing our military personnel.

Our role in personnel was to facilitate two combat-ready bomb wings as soon as possible. One wing was transferred in, and we were developing a new one. Before I left there, we had accomplished all this. Col. Travis Heatherington, one of the nicest and most professional officers I had ever met, was promoted to the rank of brigadier general and went from being a wing commander to commander of our newly formed air division.

One sad thing that happened there will always stick with me and give me sympathy for truly troubled people. Our air police squadron commander, responsible for law enforcement and security, most importantly security of weapons, I found out, was a very sick man. One of his master sergeants came to me and told me that neither he nor one of his people could approach any of the senior commanders, but he thought I could, since I worked with them, to convey that his commander needed to be relieved of his command because he was crazy, as he stated it. I told him he was nuts and what he suggested would be suicide for me. I knew Sergeant Felix well, a solid, responsible man, and concluded that if he was concerned, there probably was a problem.

After considerable thought, mind you, I was a twenty-one- or twenty-two-year-old staff sergeant being asked to warn our commanders that one of their squadron commanders was probably in need of mental health care. Lt. Col. Frank A. Taylor, the director of personnel, was a very rigid, proud professional officer; but I was closer to him, so I told him what I had been told and how irregular it was for me to come to him, but I felt there was a problem and I felt he should talk to our base commander about this.

Shortly after our conversation, the major really lost it and was sent to the psychiatric ward at Eglin Air Force Base at Fort Walton, Florida. I'd never met the major but had observed him to be a rather distant person. To my surprise sometime later, he approached my desk one day and wanted to talk. He, it seemed to me, just had to tell me what his problem was. I was surrounded by other people and wanted to protect him, so I suggested we go to another area to talk. He told me that he had had trouble before. Mind you, this was a man I don't think I had ever talked to before. Someone had to have told him about me knowing he had a problem. He went on and on about his past problems, and I remember telling him I thought he should try to get assigned to a less-stressful job and serve out his time until he could retire. At that time, an officer, who had been an officer for ten years, could finish out his time as an enlisted man and then retire as an officer, when he had served a total of twenty years. I finally coaxed him to his car, wished him well, saluted him, and never saw him again.

Lieutenant Matthews didn't change his behavior, and Colonel Taylor destroyed his career by giving him a performance report that stated that he did not run our section, because I did. He was right; I decided how and what we did, and he just signed his name where an officer's signature was required. He agreed with Colonel Taylor that I did call the shots, but even after he retired I could still tell there was some resentment toward me as he reminded me that Colonel Taylor had destroyed his career.

Again, I was surprised at the trust people put in me because of the put-downs as a child. Subsequently, as people made mistakes, I began supervising more and more supervisors, who in most cases were older than me and outranked me, after they also were demoted, until I effectively became the personnel sergeant major in charge of the personnel shop. Effectively I began working directly for the colonel as he refused to sign anything that I had not determined to be ready for his signature and had initialed.

I continued to run my section also and supervise everything in personnel except the officers' section. The pressure was so great that I beat the colonel to work and left late, but I put a stop to the improper assignments of people and other things the colonel was under severe pressure about, because so much had gone wrong on his watch.

Promotions were frozen, and I was doing a master sergeant's job, one grade lower than I was in the army, so I applied to be retrained into the weapons control systems field in order to get promoted. Colonel Taylor was a good man, and he threw a fit when I was accepted for retraining and tried to get me to cancel my new assignment, but I told him he knew how hard I worked and I just had to go so I could get ahead.

I went to Lowry Air Force Base at Denver, Colorado, for a year of school, prior to being sent to my first duty station in that job. My first assignment was at the Duluth Municipal Airport, at Duluth, Minnesota. Our fighter squadron of F-102 fighter planes had the responsibility of launching and confronting Russian bombers approaching the United States from the north.

While in Duluth, my kids, Jackie and Steven, got initiated to very cold weather. They walked to school in what seemed to Southerners as unbearable weather conditions.

It was a very bad time for me workwise as I outranked many of the people in my new world of electronic maintenance, and they resented all of us who had retrained from other jobs as we presented a threat to their future promotions. They got their revenge by giving all of us so-so performance reports.

I learned the new challenge pretty well, and in late 1959, we were all tested to see who would be selected to be trained on the digital computer that was in the weapons control system of the new F-106 aircraft we were to receive in 1960.Out of a hundred people, I was one of the five selected to be sent Los Angeles, California, to attend six months of training on the computer by the company who manufactured the new weapons system. I still comment on the fact that in the binary number system, when you add 1 and 1, I was shocked that the answer is 0—yes, zero!

The Los Angeles climate didn't agree with my sons Jackie and Steven, and they were sick a lot. Steve got a mastoid infection that was so serious that the doctor treating him thought he might never leave the hospital alive, but fortunately, he did.

I returned to Duluth and seemed to slowly grasp all that was involved this new endeavor, but I studied the technical manuals and finally learned how the computer worked and the problems that were encountered when subjecting all the electronics of a computer to the temperature changes that were encountered when an aircraft is flying into forty- and fifty-below-zero temperatures and the normal temperatures are very cold.

After we returned to Minnesota, my sons were healthier but again had to get out in the severe cold.

I was at Duluth until August of 1962, when I was transferred to Tyndall Air Force Base at Panama City, Florida. I will always remember the thirty-nine-degree temperature on the morning in August when I drove out of Duluth on my way to Florida.

A few days later, we arrived in Florida and found the heat and temperature nearly unbearable. We rented an apartment and soon enrolled Jackie and Steven in school. They walked to school there also but found the weather much more bearable and tolerated the climate much better than they did California. After we were there a few months, I bought my first house.

When I went to work, I found out that I was to take charge of the computer maintenance section of our maintenance shop. I quickly found out how badly the shop equipment and all the computer components in the roughly thirty aircraft had been maintained and set out to immediately begin improving the quality of repairs and a complete rework all the equipment in the aircraft and in the shop mock-ups where we tested computer units.

I had to bend some ears quickly about shoddy work not being acceptable, and the quality of our work brought me more favorable attention than I thought I deserved because I saw myself as just doing my job.

I stayed there for about twenty-six months, and it took about that much time to completely rework everything in all the aircraft and keep up with our flying schedule. About the time I left I received a promotion to the rank of technical sergeant, the same rank that I left the army with when I was twenty years old. I couldn't believe the outpouring of support and how pleased everyone was about my promotion. I had left personnel work because promotions were frozen and had to retrain twice in order to get to a job where promotions weren't frozen.

There was a classified project ongoing in Alaska, and I volunteered to go there and was assigned there in November 1964. I chose to drive up there and really got an introduction to traveling in severely cold weather, on a dirt road, with my wife, two sons, and a dog. We were on the road for thirteen days.

On Christmas Day of 1964, staying with my brother who was stationed there also, I had what seemed to be a heart attack and thought I really was dying. I think the ambulance crew thought I was too, from the look on their faces as they cared for me. The emergency room doctor told me later that I was the calmest one there. I told him, "Yeah, I really thought I was going to die." They told me later they thought I was lucky and had passed a small clot. It sapped my strength for a month or two, and then I was fine again. Their theory was it was caused by me sitting for thirteen days driving to Alaska.

When I got there, assuming I was going to do computer work, I was informed that I was to learn the entire weapons control system and would learn while supervising work on the aircraft. I informed the sergeant in charge of all the electronic maintenance that I was pretty cocky, but to me he was assigning me to a job I wasn't sure I could do what he expected. He turned out to be right, and I took on more supervisory responsibility until I took over all the electronic maintenance before I left there.

The last year I was there my commander called me each morning at 0630, and we planned where we would send aircraft to that day. As a detachment with limited aircraft, equipment, and people, we did what we had to do to get the job done. He had one officer who didn't know what he was doing, so he and I effectively ran the place. I felt good about the fact that I always managed to give him an aircraft that would do the job electronically. He and I became about as close and confident in each other's ability as I've ever seen between an officer and an enlisted man. I really respected him, and I think he felt the same way about me.

I left Alaska in June 1968 and went to Selfridge Air Force Base, near Detroit, Michigan. I felt as though I didn't really have a job there, as being a computer technician and maintenance shop shift supervisor was like not having a job compared to my responsibility in Alaska.

My first two sons, Jack Jr. and Steve, were teenagers at that time, and I worked with them in the Boy Scouts as I had done some in Alaska as time permitted. I met my new commander, Lt. Col. Euel Wainwright, during this time and thought nothing about it at the time. I had not been there long until I learned that my successor in Alaska had to be fired because he could not get the job done. It didn't enhance your career when you couldn't keep four aircraft on alert at two different sites twenty-four hours each day. The aircraft at the alert sites had to be airborne in five minutes when an unknown aircraft crossed our border from Russia. The air force headquarters at the Pentagon took a failure to get the job done there very seriously. The fact that I did well there made me look good in the eyes of our senior commanders.

My last assignment was a transfer with the 94th Fighter Interceptor Squadron from Selfridge to Wurtsmith Air Force Base, Michigan. While there on March 8, 1970, my third son, William L. Pusch, was born. I didn't know at the time what an impact he would have on my life. I was mostly a computer technician and night shift supervisor of our electronic maintenance shop. Colonel Wainwright (no relation to Gen. Jonathan Wainwright) treated me as though I were an equal, to the point it bothered me as I had a very professional boss whom he would ignore. He would come to the shop, and a lot of times he would bring someone he was with over and introduce me to them as Jack Pusch, never by rank. I was a master sergeant and thought this strange. I later thought about that and told Bill that I thought he really looked at me as being someone more qualified than my rank indicated.

Late in the year 1970, Colonel Wainwright would call me about the status of an item we were working on and would believe me and not trust what his chief of maintenance and others had told him. He was selected for promotion from lieutenant colonel to colonel (one step under a brigadier general). Embarrassingly soon after his selection, our unit failed an operational readiness inspection (ORI). I was advised that I had been selected by Colonel Wainwright to take charge of the night maintenance shift of the electronics equipment on the aircraft. I blew my lid but was told by our electronics maintenance officer that he selected me because he knew I was responsible and really cared about what happened.

I did what I was told and as we had real problems, I saw the colonel a lot, and he would ask my opinion about some things I really knew little about, but he always seemed so side with me if someone else had a different opinion.

One day, one of my master sergeant friends asked me if the colonel and I were homosexuals. When I asked him what brought that about, he laughed and said because the colonel would always listen to me and not others. I really was as puzzled about that as he was.

As in Alaska, I was doing a job I had never really been trained for, but I let it be known that the only thing I would accept was to do the job right the first time. It didn't take too long to get the maintenance up to the level that we passed the next ORI and got the colonel off the hook.

Many years later, I told my Bill that I thought the reason the colonel treated me the way he did and trusted my judgment when he was in trouble was that he and my former boss, in Alaska, another good colonel, had to have talked about me. Colonels in Colonel Wainwright's position are usually very serious, no-nonsense people. And he was. I told Bill that I thought the reason he treated me as he did was that he thought I deserved to be much higher in rank. He never called me sergeant; I was always Jack Pusch when he talked to me or about me to others, I was told.

Shortly after I got him out of trouble, it was time to retire and I went to see the colonel and we had our final talk. I told him he was going to be a general, which he tried to brush off, but I told him he and people in leadership positions had to really improve the behavior of our enlisted people. Morale among them was low, and they had become very undisciplined.

The last time I knew what he was doing, he was a major general. He later died of a heart attack.

I always felt good that my final years in the air force were trying times and that I had the trust and respect so many senior officers.

I moved my family back to the home I owned in Panama City, Florida, in November of 1970, to begin my new life as a civilian.

CHAPTER 4
My Father

My father, Edwin Kurt Pusch, came to the United States from Wilbaddungen, Germany. I do not know much about his early time here, but I do know that he had come to the United States when he was sixteen for a visit to an uncle in Kansas, and he told me that he decided during that visit that he was coming back the next year and he was not going to go back to Germany. World War I was about to start and he was supposed to become an officer in the German army and he said he had no desire to be in the German army under any circumstances. I think it was in 1917 that he came back and stayed here. He announced his decision to not return to Germany on the second visit and immediately was disowned. He said his action ended for all time his further communications with any of his family. Therefore, I know nothing about his family.

Not able to speak English, he said he did whatever he could to make enough money to live. How it happened, I do not know, but he learned English and became a print newsman and owned a few small newspapers, he said. He was married once before he married my mother, but I know very little about that marriage. The one thing all who knew him saw was his character. He was so generous; he helped a lot of people who took advantage of him. That is one reason I had to help support him the last few years of his life. He told me we all should not lie, steal, or do anything wrong, and to treat every woman like a lady whether she was or not.

When he married my mother, he tried to help my grandparents and wound up supporting them for the rest of their lives. They had once been wealthy, but my grandfather was, according to my grandmother, a mean man who had once killed someone and became a drunk and lost everything long before my dad married my mother.

My father came to Russellville, Arkansas, in the late '20s, I figure, and married my mother, Allene Anderson. He was working as Linotype operator for the Courier-Democrat. She was much younger than he was, I estimate, by twenty to twenty-five years. She was living at home with her parents, Mr. and Mrs. L. D. Anderson in Russellville.

Little do I know about the circumstances, but my father got a job in Oklahoma and moved there; and I was told by an uncle, my mother's brother, Burford, that my father moved the Andersons to Oklahoma also, trying to get my grandfather to sober up. That didn't work, and my grandparents moved back to 411 North Jonesboro Avenue, in Russellville. After my mother died, we went to live with the Andersons in Russellville.

The one thing I noticed after he came to live with me in the country was that all who got to know him there thought highly of him, and in one case, the person told me he literally hated my grandfather. He said he so despised him because he was so mean to my brother and me.

CHAPTER 5
My Mother

I have no memory of my mother. She died when I was about twenty-two months old. I remember the Andersons talking about what a good person she was.

She was buried in Russellville, about five miles from where we lived, but the Andersons lost track of where her grave was.

When I was young, I tried to find her grave but never could. During my search, many people told me what a sweet, kind person she was. People had died, and those still alive could not be sure which unmarked grave was hers.

As I got older, I could not envision losing the grave of someone, a child, a sweet person like she was known to be. I always blamed the Andersons as they lived so close to the cemetery for about two or three years after she died. The one I blame the most is her brother Burford as he owned a car and lived in Russellville. My dad was off working and supporting the Andersons and my brother and me, so I really blame him the least.

For years I kept trying to find people who had known her and had attended her funeral, but I finally had to give up my search for her grave. After I gave up on ever finding her grave, I looked up as many people who had known her as I could find, and many would tell me about the good things she had done and said. From what people told me, my son Bill, whom I lost on January 7, 2005, must have gotten a lot of his kindness from her.

CHAPTER 6
My Return to Civilian Life

After I retired from the air force in 1971, I moved my family back to Panama City, Florida, as I owned a home there that I had bought in 1963.

Bill was about a year old and I didn't want to travel and be away from him. I had traveled enough. His brothers Jackie and Steven were respectively about fourteen and fifteen years old at that time. They graduated from high school there and were out on their own after the normal teenage part-time jobs, dating, and all that go with those years, leaving Bill the only child at home.

I went to work for Sears and thought I would work another twenty years and retire. Bill adjusted to the move well, and I really enjoyed him. I had a lot across the street from our home and decided that it would become a good garden spot. I had a trench dug halfway from each side and halfway between front and back in order to put an irrigation system in. I put posts in to support sprinklers, mounted about five feet high in order to water the entire garden. When I ran the plastic hose in the trenches and made all the connections, I had Bill with me, and at the end of the day, he at approximately the age of one and a half or two years old looked like a little black boy as he was covered with dirt. That was quite a change for me as I had not been that patient with my first two boys, unknown to me that signaled quite a change as all Bill's life we liked to be together.

I had a lot of responsibility during my military service and Sears saw how aggressive I was and they placed me in charge of their furniture department. I ran it like it was mine and grew the business to the point that I knew I would be better off running my own store and planned to do so. I made them more money than anyone ever had before. Before I left Sears, I injured my back for the fourth time and never got over it.

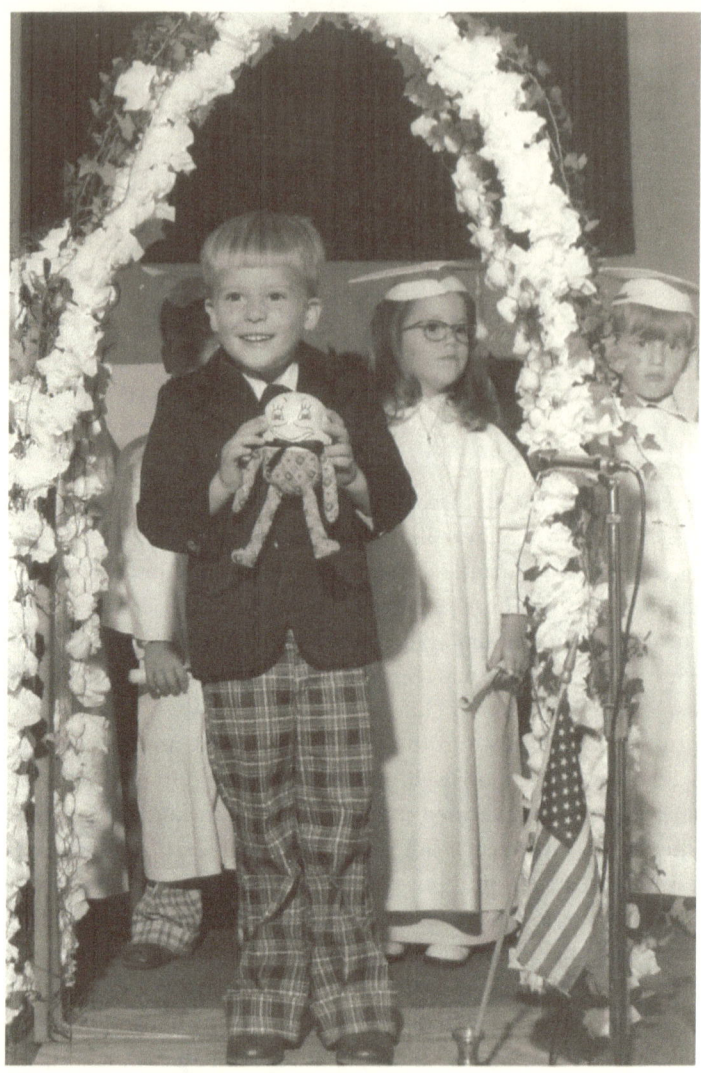

Bill at 3 yrs old, in pre-school, 1973

Bill had started to preschool there when he was still a baby, but it was apparent to all that knew him just how he stood out among his peers by his personality and behavior. He was a very bright child, his father's pride and joy, and was loved by all who came to know him. What really stood out about him was his caring attitude, his will to do what was right, and always being so respectful to all he was around.

The humidity in Florida was aggravating my back condition, so in 1977, I moved back to Arkansas, where I had bought property in 1975, anticipating going into business for myself. The ten acres I had bought was out in the country from Russellville. I built a house there and wondered how I was ever going to raise Bill with a back that kept me in the bed a lot.

How it came about, I don't know, but I decided I could invest in the stock market whether I could go or not. I read everything the library had and watched business news until I bought my first stock, and with God's help, I made mostly all good choices and got on my feet financially.

I had rarely attended church, but we joined the Church of Christ in Dover. Shortly afterward, the church wanted me to head a building committee. I reluctantly agreed to do so, and the goal was to add thirty-six hundred square feet of classroom space and to add a bedroom to the parsonage. All went well until one day, I learned the pastor and a deacon had taken it on themselves to do some additional work that had not been approved. Being church business, I thought if that was the way church people did things, it was time for me to resign, which I did. They wanted to borrow two hundred thousand dollars at 17 percent interest, which I knew the church could never pay off. After I left, they only borrowed fifty thousand dollars and completed what was originally planned, and they had a hard time paying that off. Bill said one of the long-time members came to him one day and told him that the stand I took about what the church should do was the right one. After I left the church, Bill's mother continued to take Bill to church there, which I will always be grateful to her for as it started his strong lifetime belief in God.

In my early years, I had never seriously thought that much about being a Christian. When my son Steven got so sick with the mastoid problem while I was attending computer school in 1960, I began praying each night, and fortunately he got well. Every night after that, I prayed for those in need, and the Lord's Prayer before I became a Christian.

After my experience in the Dover church, I was very disillusioned that a preacher and a deacon would act like that, even though the pastor agreed he had done wrong. I didn't become a member of another church for about fifteen years.

Bill had always been kind and was loved by everyone. I knew he had a good heart, and I knew he was in for an awakening when he discovered that not all people are that way.

In about 1986, my aunt Louise who lived in Kansas had to be placed in a nursing home. I was down with my chronic back problem and couldn't go, but Bill and his mother along with my brother and his wife went up there to help get her moved. While there, Bill met Frank Dare, who had grown up with us on Shinn Mountain. When Bill came home, he was furious. He said Frank had told him how the Andersons had ridiculed and put me down when I was a kid. He asked me why I put flowers on their graves after the way I had been treated. I told him they were my mother's parents and I understood their bitterness, to some extent. They had once been wealthy, and now they were humiliated by the fact that later they depended on my father for their very existence.

Bill went to school in Dover, about five miles from where we lived, and was a joy to raise and see him grow up. He was loved by everyone. He loved living in the country. When he graduated from high school, I wanted him to begin college and get his degree in mathematics. He told me he had been in school all his life and he wanted to go into the army for two years as the army bonus would pay for his math degree. He was correct about being in school so long as he had started to preschool while he was only three years old. I understood how he felt about school and agreed to his choice of entering the army.

By this time, his mother and I had divorced, ending thirty-three years of arguments over spending money and disagreements over how both the mother and the father had a role in deciding how family life should be conducted, not just the mother, as her mother had done.

Bill got his private pilot's license in 1986, and as soon as he qualified, he told me to "come on"; we were going flying. We flew over the local area and our home. There was an article in the local paper about him and how he was referred to as the singing pilot. He said it was boring going from town to town, so he sang a lot. Flying was his first love.

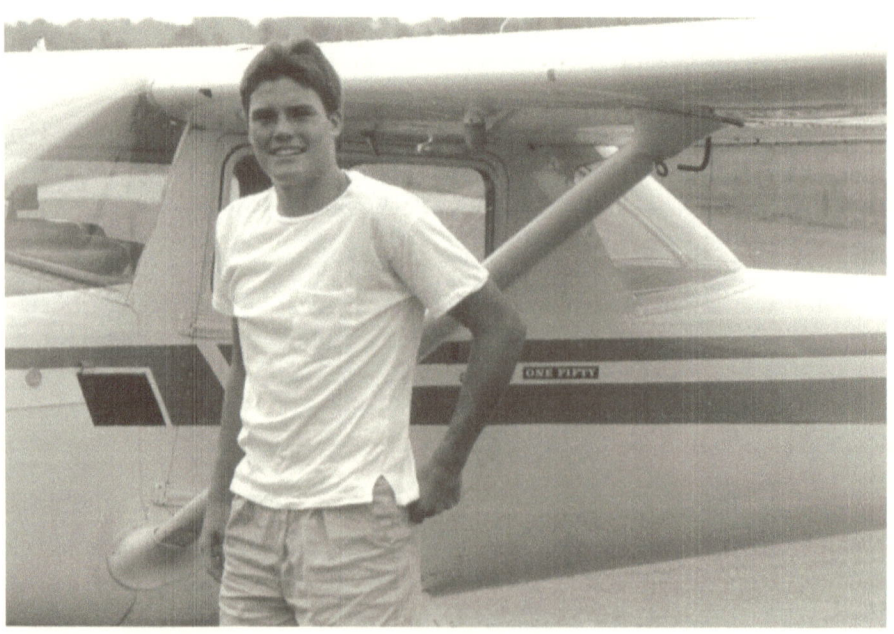

Bill at 16 yrs old, the day he got his private pilot's license, 1986

We lived near Dover, but a lot of Bill's friends lived in Russellville. One who has been special all these years was Drew Crumpler. Drew's dad, Joe Crumpler, was a well-known and well-loved surgeon in Russellville. The first time Drew came to our house, I told Drew he was OK but he needed to get his dad to fix the hole in his ear. Bill told me Drew only wore the earring to aggravate Joe. I fussed at Drew like I did with Bill, but he once told me I was the only adult he could talk to, and I told him I might have been a kid once. He and Bill and I would do things together from time to time, and I got to meet Joe and Drew's mother, Faye. I soon learned that Bill was in good hands at the Crumplers, and I think they felt the same way when Drew was with Bill and me. Faye looked after Bill like he was her child.

If I needed anything done, I could always count on Bill and Drew to do it and do it right. Sometimes I express my confidence in Drew's ability to handle something and he asks why I'm so confident in his ability and I tell him I've been watching him since he was a kid and I know what he can do.

I bought Bill his first vehicle in the fall of 1986, a little Mazda pickup. He was so well grounded by that time; he wanted a truck with a burgundy interior, and he waited so he could get the color he wanted, a grey exterior also.

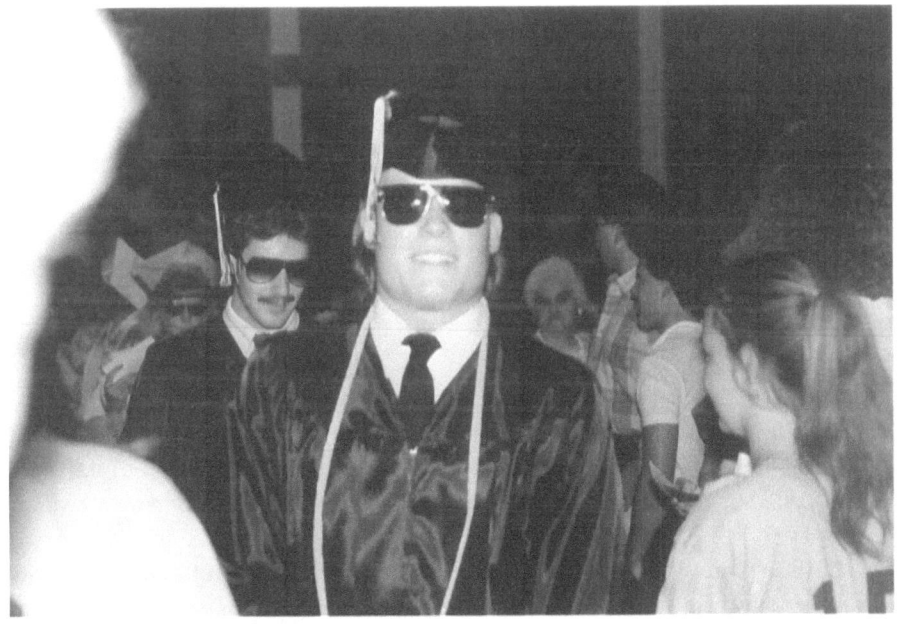

Bill's High School Graduation, 1988

Bill was assigned to the 101st Airborne Division, at Fort Campbell, Kentucky. My son, so intelligent as a private in the U.S. Army, made no sense to me, but we had become so close that I knew he had time to get his education and do well in life. He called a lot and came home every chance he had, which was quite often. I got to know the names of many people he had met, and we had many good discussions about his new life. He told me he really missed our time to talk more than anything with us being separated, but we made up for it as much as we could.

Drew missed Bill as much as I did, and he would call to see if I needed him to assist me with anything and see if I had heard from Bill. I often thought about how thoughtful Drew was and the fact that at that young age he was so kind and considerate.

Shortly before Bill's two years in the army was finished, it was discovered he had histoplasmosis, a fungus in his right lung. Faye told me she didn't want just any doctor operating on Bill and said she thought Joe should talk to the surgeon to see if he knew what he was doing. I agreed, and Joe called the doctor and told me he was satisfied the doctor knew what he was doing.

It looked like cancer on his X-rays, but the first thing his surgeon told me was that "It's not cancer" and proceeded to tell me what he had discovered and what he did, which was to remove the lower lobe of Bill's right lung. Since Bill had his pilot's license, I told him Bill loved to fly and was concerned how the surgery would affect that, and he told me he was so healthy that his lung would expand and he would be fine.

After the surgery, he was in a lot of pain, a lot of cutting for lung surgery. One of the army corpsmen told me he was asking for morphine too often; he was really torn about what to do. Neither of us wanted him to become morphine dependent, so I told him Bill was my baby but he had a low tolerance for pain. I told him to just wait a little longer between shots and that would solve the problem. He did, and everything worked out well.

Unknown to me, Bill had decided to go to Fort Rucker, Alabama, to learn to fly helicopters, and it was during the physical examination that the histoplasmosis was discovered.

I did not want him in military service after his goal of going to the naval academy had not worked out. I saw his ability as being too great to be just another military officer whose advancement in rank would be limited short of having a military academy education. For this reason, I wanted him to pursue a civilian career.

I have so many precious memories of Bill, but one stands out. A few days after the surgery, he was very inactive because of the pain, but doing well, I asked him if it would be OK for me to go home; and without opening his eyes, he slowly shook his head, no. My daredevil, not afraid of Satan himself, wasn't ready for his pop to leave him yet.

He was sent home to recuperate for thirty days. I was living in an apartment in Russellville, waiting to build a house in Russellville. Drew was with us a lot, and one night Bill and Drew were having a few beers and I saw Bill had had enough and I told Bill not to drink anymore. He told me he was twenty years old, and I told him I didn't care how old he was; he was not drinking any more. He listened to me reluctantly. Drew later asked me if I wasn't being a little too hard on Bill, and I told him no; Bill had just had serious surgery, and he had drunk enough.

With a bad back, I didn't need to be out in the country, so I built the house in Russellville, and Bill and I were close to Arkansas Tech University, where he got his math degree after coming home from the army. Being as dedicated to our country as he was though he convinced the army to take him back during Operation Desert Storm, which I opposed, but fortunately he was sent to Hawaii and not to Iraq. This caused him to lose a semester in college, but he said it was his duty to serve our country. I was proud of him, but I felt that with the lung surgery he had given enough, as the army thought that sleeping in an old chicken house during his army service had caused the histoplasmosis.

While attending Tech, Bill went to work part-time for Keith Shipley, who had done the plumbing, heat and air and electrical work for me when I built my house. He said he and Keith talked about the Bible as much as he did about work. Keith was an extremely devout Christian, and I will always be grateful to him for his good influence on Bill.

I am not really sure of the time frame, but while attending Tech, he also worked at the Blue Chip Ice company for some time. They wanted him to go to work for them full-time, but I told him to not limit his advancement by going with a small company. My thinking was, a management job in a small company didn't offer the long-time job security he needed, and I knew his potential was for far greater responsibility.

While attending Tech, Bill met Lisa Harwell, and later I found out she said she was going to marry him before he even knew her. She was a sweet girl, and she was good enough for my son (several other girls had not been, Dad was picky). They would go to church on Sunday and I would cook lunch for them and we'd eat and then they'd go do their thing. They had a quick marriage by a justice of the peace, on September 5, 1992, unknown to me, just hours before Drew and his fiancée Jeanette got married, which of course Bill, Lisa, and I attended. They had a formal marriage ceremony later, but Bill said no way was Drew going to get married before he did!

Bill and his Lambda Chi Alpha fraternity brothers really kept up with each other, and they and their families got together as often as they could. Bill and Lisa, Layton and Robin Lee, Robert and Stephanie Young, Carmen and Heath Stump, Brad and Melanie Thresher, John and Amber Reidel, and J. J. and Heather Pitman, and their families, would all get together in Yellville, Arkansas, each spring beginning in May of 1996, ending with 2003, camping and canoeing down the Buffalo River.

Brad Thresher recently told me about an incident when Alexa became curious about a tent rope during one of those outings and was examining it when Bill went over to her and explained the function of the rope in holding the tent up. He said normally it was us men's thing to tell her to just get away and leave the rope alone, but Bill didn't do that; he took the time to explain to her the purpose of the rope.

Brad said he learned things like that from Bill that he used later in raising his kids.

That was my Bill, always the good, caring father.

He and Lisa gave me Alexa Pusch on May13, 1993, as my third grandchild. My son Steven had given me my first, Steven Pusch, Jr., on September 27, 1986, and Angela on February 13, 1988, whom I have only seen a few times. With Alexa, however, it has been altogether different; I've been around her since she was born, as well as James Benjamen, her brother who was born on July 11, 1998.

They moved into an apartment, and I bought them a washer and dryer, which I think Lisa still has. Lisa was going to college to become a teacher, and Bill was going to get his math degree. Bill was a proud father, and both he and Lisa were wonderful parents. If Lisa was concerned about Alexa, she would call me from time to time and see if I thought she should take her to the doctor. No one could have been made more proud to have her as my son's wife and the mother of my grandchild. The same is true today.

They joined the Second Baptist Church in Russellville and became very active in the church. Bill had been baptized in the Church of Christ, and Lisa had been baptized in the Methodist Church. When they joined Second Baptist, they were simultaneously baptized by their new preacher, David Mclemore.

I was very proud of both of them when the church did a play about young couples' marriage challenges. They played the young mother and father. The church decided to invite the public and charged ten dollars per adult for admission. I was pleasantly surprised at how well they played their roles and how many people attended.

Around the time Bill got his math degree, it was discovered he had type 1 diabetes. I cried when I learned this, and Bill said, "Dad, it could be cancer." He and I talked about his future, and he reminded me again that his diabetes could have been cancer, so it wasn't all that bad. Diabetes put an end to his flying, so we discussed his future, and he decided to go to law school. When I first mentioned law school to Bill, I couldn't have been prouder of him than when he looked me in the eye and asked if he could be a lawyer and live the life we believed in. My reply was "Yes, just stay away from the crooks." His question was prompted by what my dad had taught me—you don't lie, cheat, steal, or do wrong; and you treat every woman like she is a lady whether she is or not.

Their truck, which I had bought for Bill when he was a junior in high school, was about to be worn out. I told Lisa the truck would not make it through law school, and we decided another truck would be best for them, so Bill and I got together and I bought him a new Ford Ranger truck. They moved to Little Rock in July of 1995 so he could start attending law school in the fall of 1995.

In August of 1996, I joined the First Baptist Church in Russellville. I was pleasantly surprised to see so many Christians who acted like Christians. I was particularly impressed that so many doctors and dentists there would close or reduce their practices and go to Africa for a week or two each year and treat the poor people there. Our pastor, Dr. Stephen Davis, was a very dedicated man and took his job very seriously. He was there for all the people, wealthy or poor. He is one of my heroes in life.

I had attended a few Pentecostal churches from time to time, and I saw and heard about behavior that I couldn't believe anyone claiming to be a Christian would be a part of. My thought was, surely, people calling themselves Christians don't act like this. My uncle Burford had been a member of one of those churches for years and told stories that convinced me that yes, some of them really do act that way. All of that made me especially proud of my church.

Law school was tough for Bill and Lisa financially. Lisa got a job at the KinderCare Learning Center for two years and then began teaching at Fair Park Elementary School beginning in September of 1997. Bill was so busy at school that he had little time to work. He worked in the legal section at the state department of finance and administration as much as he could. He went to summer school also and graduated in three and a half years. The state wanted him to go to work for them, but he said he needed more money than the state could pay.

Bill was so independent that he was determined to make his own way in life regardless of how tough it was.

I found out he was wearing an old parka to law school and bought him a nice Columbia nylon multipurpose jacket that he could wear under multiple weather conditions. I knew he had to be embarrassed about his old jacket, but he was so proud and independent he would not tell me he needed a new jacket. That and the fact he put $50 each month into a mutual fund showed his maturity beyond his years. I recently asked Lisa if she still had the jacket I bought him, and she does. A jacket that symbolizes what kind of good, decent, and self-reliant man he was.

CHAPTER 7
Bill, the Lawyer

Bill went to work for the Rochelle law firm in early 1998. The bulk of his work seemed to be defending school teachers for the Arkansas Education Association. He also did work for those who had all types of legal problems.

One of the first things I noticed was how he got involved in his clients' problems, and being so kindhearted, he would wind up working his heart out for them and in several cases never getting paid. I told him I was glad he was so kindhearted, but he must remember how much law school cost and have his clients pay their bills like he did. He learned in time and just wrote off some billing he came to know he would never collect.

I talked to Mr. Rochelle and told him Bill would in time make him a good lawyer, and I was informed that Bill was already a good lawyer. He had not been there long before he won a seventy-five-thousand-dollar suit he had filed, and Mr. Rochelle reminded me of that.

That he was making a pretty good salary by that time he and Lisa purchased their house, in Cammack Village, a little town, surrounded by Little Rock. It was a cute little house, and they were proud of their first home. Lisa painted and really fixed up the interior, and they really enjoyed it. Bill surprised me by really being more of a handyman than I thought he was capable of. I was really proud of both of them.

Bill was active in the community and was appointed to the position of city attorney and ran for another term and was elected. He served out that term and lost the next election. I was really glad he did as he was really too busy at his regular job and Dad thought he was working too much, having diabetes.

While working there, he met Dale Whitney, who was a policeman. Dale was later made the chief of police, and Bill and Lisa became good friends with Torrie (Dale's wife) and daughter Sydney. Their friendship grew, and he and Dale did a lot together.

Bill stayed at Rochelle for about two years and grew unhappy with some of the unethical practices he saw used by some lawyers. He would call me and start talking about a case that I could tell was really bothering him. Once, he called and I could tell the other lawyer was trying to take advantage of his kindness and I told him to tell the other one that the talking was over and they would settle it in court. Later, he called and said the other attorney sent him a check to settle out of court. He learned that some people don't even pay their lawyers, and he started making his client pay a little up front before he would take their case.

CHAPTER 8

Bill, the Businessman

Needing more money and preferring to practice business law, he applied for and was hired by Acxiom Corporation, a data company, in Little Rock, in the summer of 2000.

I'm certainly not familiar with all he did there, but he did a lot of business contracts. There, like in his first job as a lawyer, he never told me anything that would identify clients or details of what he was doing, but he would tell me about run-ins with other lawyers whose methods he didn't like and how he came to understand that you have to take a firm position and stick with it.

Because of his intelligence and personality, he was chosen to brief the senior corporate leaders from time to time.

While there, he said he would be given unsettled legal situations to resolve on several occasions. He said he would tell the opposing attorneys sometimes to come off their hard stand and listen to common sense and apparently resolved several long-standing cases.

He liked his work but needed more money, so he said he told them he was looking for a job that paid more, and he said they in turn would tell him they couldn't afford to lose him.

He and his good friend from his Army National Guard and reserve service, Roy Minton, took Microsoft tests that qualified them for good-paying jobs in the data field. BMC Software in Houston, Texas, was going to hire both of them for sixty-five thousand dollars a year based on the certification they had achieved. I did not want Bill to accept the job, as it required worldwide travel, because of his diabetes. He listened to me and did not accept it, but Roy did and stayed with them a few years and quit because of all the traveling he had to do.

Roy became a member of MENSA and after Bill's death I asked him why Bill didn't and he said Bill had no interest in taking the examination. I think Bill would have passed the MENSA examination also, but he just wasn't interested in things like that. He just saw himself as no more intelligent than anyone else.

While at Acxiom, his abilities became very apparent with time, and they sent him to San Diego, California, for a few days to see if he could clear up what apparently had been a communications problem. While there, he went to the officers' club at a Marine Corps base. Did he ever have some stories to tell me when he went home. He told about meeting a Marine Corps major whose life had been by saved by the 101st Airborne Division. This was where Bill had served during his two years in the army. He said the major got up and saluted him, and Bill was surprised as he was just a captain. He said he questioned the major about why he did that, and the major said had it not been for the 101st, he would not have been alive then.

He said later that his boss told him they had had a problem of long standing with the San Diego office and he had taken care of the problem during his short visit there.

With his personality, he was warmly received by everyone who ever met him. It was easy for him to get people on the right track.

He said one of the managers there expressed his dislike for lawyers frequently. He said this guy told him he was the only lawyer he had ever seen who knew how business operated. He said this guy told him that he had informed the senior leaders that if Bill left it would hurt the company, but they did not offer him any more money, until he was leaving.

That went on for some time, and after he had been there for about three years, he got a call from a fraternity brother, Brad Thresher, telling him that he had recommended him for a job at an Arvest Bank that had a problem that really needed cleaned up quickly.

He went for the interview, and they wanted him immediately, but he said wouldn't just walk out and would give Acxiom two weeks' notice of his departure. Another instance of doing the right thing and his dad was really proud that he thought that way. Arvest agreed to hire him with a 50 percent pay raise and move him to the new location. Acxiom wanted to match what Arvest had agreed to pay him, but he said he had given his word and he was going. Dad was again proud of his high principles.

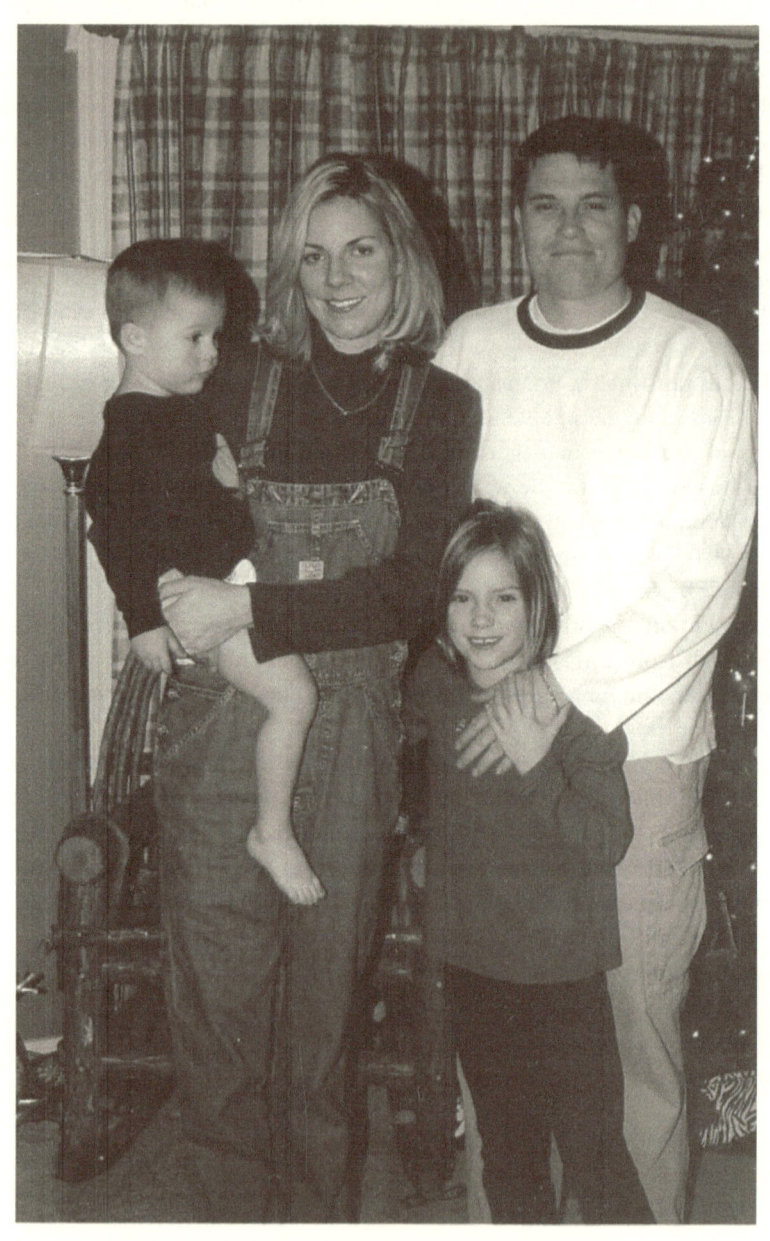

Bill, Lisa, Alexa and Ben, Christmas 2000

CHAPTER 9
Bill in Banking

As agreed, he reported to the Arvest in Yellville, Arkansas, on July 28, 2003, as the Special Asset Manager.

The problem he was hired to correct was a large number of loans had fallen into default status, and it was his job to somehow turn repossessed cars, homes, vacant land, businesses, and whatever into as much money as he possible could.

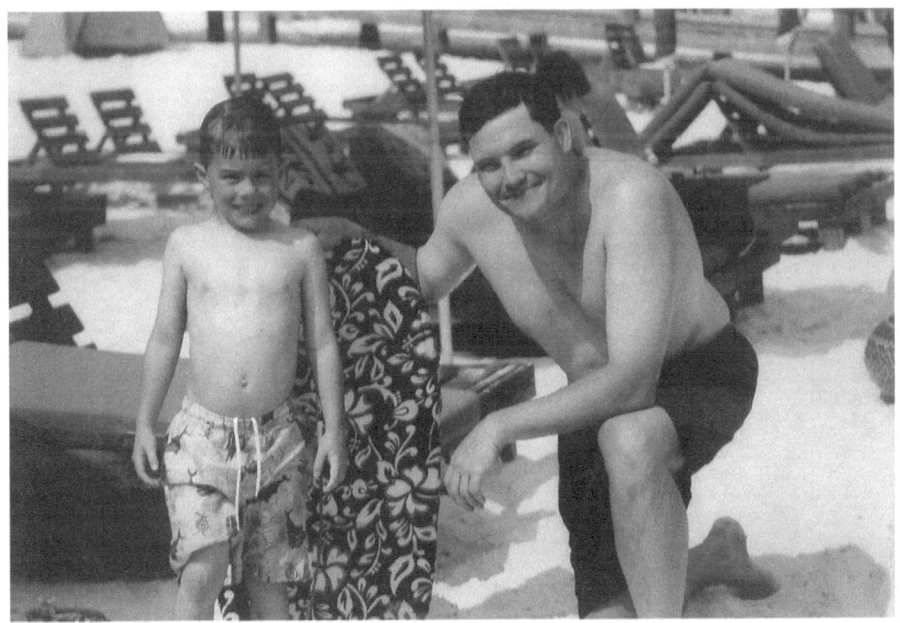

Bill and his son Ben on the beach, Gulf Shores Alabama, 2003

I don't think he realized the enormity of the problem he had been hired to clean up until he had been there awhile because he moved out of his nice office to the second floor where his people were doing the work.

We had talked a lot about how to analyze a problem and work out an approach to resolve it. I was proud of the way he formed a team of people and assigned a car man, etc., to cover most areas but handled all real estate and businesses himself. I was somewhat concerned about how he would manage his people and approach this as this really was his first time to manage a team of people, but he did it well. He began to talk about Jim Walton, as Jim, and I reminded him Jim was a billionaire, and he said, "Dad, I talk to Jim just like I talk to you." He said the first time he met Jim, he called him Mr. Walton, and Jim said, "It's Jim." Jim is the owner and chief executive officer of Arvest Bank, and the bank was one that Arvest had recently purchased.

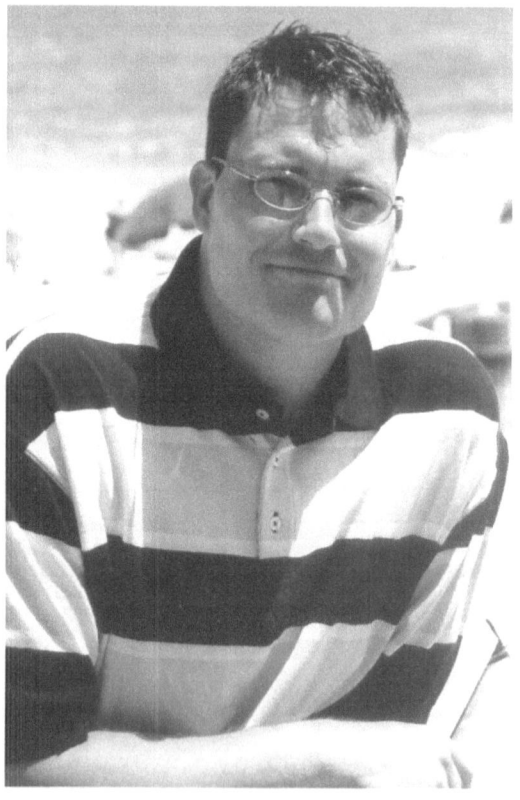

Bill as he really was, Gulf Shores Alabama, 2003

He said he asked Jim during one of Jim's visits to the bank if there was a specific way to do the job, and he said Jim told him to just do what worked best for him. He said he told Jim that he had decided to follow the system an Oklahoma bank used.

As time went on, I could tell he was getting a good handle on solving problems there. As when he was practicing law, he would start telling me something, and I knew the unstated question was "Dad, is this the right approach, or what do you think?" He called me a lot of times in the middle of the night, and had done so for a long time. I would tell him about my handling of specific situations and why I took the approach I did. When I thought it necessary, I would tell him about the unforeseen things that could occur and what to do in the event they happened. I was proud of his loyalty to Arvest and to his previous employers as he always kept company policy out of our conversations.

Bill really wanted to believe that everyone was as honest as he was. When trying to get people to pay something on their loans, he was surprised at the things they said. He said, "Dad, they will just look you in the eye and lie to you," and I would say, "Welcome to the world." It was there at Arvest that he began to see just how rotten some people are. I was somewhat like him in wanting to believe that everyone was basically honest but, like him, came to understand that a dollar will bring out the worst possible behavior in some people.

Over time, he began to make noticeable progress, and the statistics showed it. He would tell me how he had learned if his approach was working or not and how he changed procedures if he had to. I think his superiors were as pleased as I was about how quickly he got a handle on the problems and the correct solutions to handling them. I had found in life that many people cannot put their finger on the solution to a problem. I had replaced a lot of them who couldn't. He could.

As he made progress in lowering the percentage of bad loans, he would tell me about his and Jim's conversations as Jim visited the bank. I asked him what they talked about. He said they discussed business, of course, but they talked about their flying and other things they did. I was always impressed that he felt so at ease talking to Jim. He told me that his hiring was prompted by Jim's unhappiness over the problem he was hired to clean up. To me, I felt here was a lot of Sam, Jim's father, in him. It went along with some of what I'd told Bill about people, that some of the nicest people I'd known were some of the most successful.

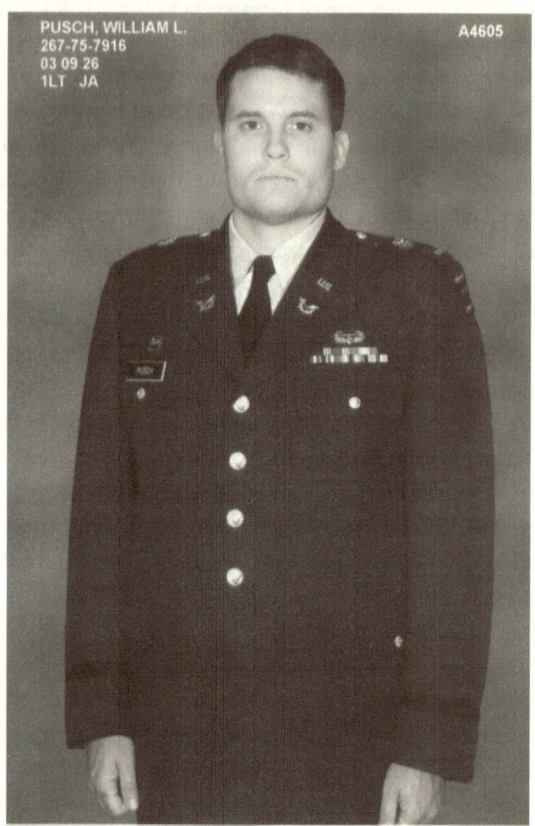

PUSCH, WILLIAM L.
267-75-7916
03 09 26
1LT   JA

A4605

Bill serving in the Army, 1ˢᵗ Lieutenant—JAG Corps, 2003

Bill got the rate of bad loans pretty low, and he said his boss, Tom Dame, told him that if he got the percentage down to, I believe, 1.5 percent by a certain time, Tom would dress up like a woman and sing him a country love song at their next meeting. My mister, serious when need be, had a fun-loving side that few at the bank apparently knew about. He said that he bought a package of panty hose and threw them on Tom's desk and told him to start getting dressed. He did better than expected, and I understand Tom did what he promised.

It took him about a year and a half to pretty well correct most of what he had been hired to do. He needed a challenge, so he said he was in Fayetteville one day and went to Scott Grigsby's office and told him that he had pretty well accomplished what he had been hired to do and he needed more money. Scott usually accompanied Jim when he visited the bank. He said the next time Scott came by the bank, by himself, and told him that they were looking for a position to move him into.

Unfortunately, on January 7, 2005, Bill had gone into Mountain Home, before going home, and on his way home he had a wreck that took his life.

He was a captain in the U.S. Army JAG Corps and was to come to my home in Little Rock that night so he could report to Camp Robinson in North Little Rock the next day for his monthly weekend duty there.

He would normally call me or I would call him before he left home, and we would have our usual chat about him eating enough so his blood sugar would not get too low during his drive to Little Rock. Usually I would wait for his arrival, and we would go out to eat.

That night we had not talked, and Lisa called very upset, telling me there had been a wreck and was told it was bad and for me to come now.

I drove to Mountain Home, praying that he was alive. Unfortunately, that was not the case I found out when I got there. She wouldn't call me while I was driving, and I think I really knew what I was going to learn once I got there, so I didn't call until I got there. The first thing I thought about was that he and I could never talk again. He told me many times how much our long talks meant to him, and he was the only one in my family that had interests similar to mine. I called their home from the Walmart parking lot in Mountain Home, and his pastor David Johnson and someone else came to get me and drove me to their home.

When I got to their house, I hugged Lisa and Alexa, and we cried harder than I had ever cried. I cried until I seemed to lose my breath and then cried again. I'll never forget what I said, "How are you supposed to deal with this?" Someone had taken Ben home with them, so I did not see him until the next day. I could not sleep and got up and drove around, which was something I had always done when bothered by something.

Somehow we got through the next few days. The night of January 10, we had visitation at the funeral home in Mountain Home. There, I met many of his new friends and talked to his pastor a long time.

One couple, Bill and Trieneke Self, came looking for me as I was visiting with Bill's pastor. We talked a long time, and I was told how much Bill had talked about me. Trieneke later did everything she could to see that I got counseling, which I did, and they will always be special people to me. At the funeral, Bill sang "It Is Well with My Soul," which, unknown to me, was my Bill's favorite hymn.

We decided to bury him in Russellville, where Bill had grown up and where he and Lisa went to college.

The funeral was at the Second Baptist Church, which Bill and Lisa had attended and been very active in church activities. Bill loved the military life so well that we had a military funeral. I retired from military service, and I remarked later that I had never seen so many military officers in my life crying. When I saw Bill's good friend and boss, Maj. Matt Ramsey, he looked at me through his tears and said, "I can't talk either."

Bill's former pastor, Dr. John Gerlach, in Little Rock, came back from Midland, Texas, to do his funeral. Major Ramsey conducted the military portion of the service and through his tears told about his first meeting Bill and how they had become best friends. The funeral lasted two and a half hours as so many people wanted to talk about him. Several talked about Bill being responsible for them having the good jobs they had. The church and parking were so packed that some left because they could not find a place to park.

We had so many people at the cemetery that friends would keep coming to me to tell me that someone was waiting to see me as soon as I could see them. An army colonel waited for his turn to tell me how much Bill was respected and cared for by his fellow officers and enlisted personnel. I believe the colonel was the only officer there who wasn't crying. I don't believe I have ever seen so many people attend a cemetery service.

After the service, R. C. Lewis, a childhood friend, told me how long the service lasted and how he was impressed at how many people had come from the area where Bill worked to attend his service. He and Lisa were loved by a lot of people. That was shown by the large discount by the funeral home and six months' free rent Lisa got from their landlord. People came to know what wonderful people Bill and Lisa were.

My only regret has been that he always wanted me with him on Christmas Day and I wasn't there for his last Christmas. I was there in 2003. He wanted to come and get me, but I didn't feel like going. Of course, I didn't know what was going to happen a couple of weeks later. One of Lisa's grandmothers died on Christmas Day and the last time I saw him alive was on December 30, 2004, about 9:00 PM or 10:00 PM, when they stopped by to see me on their way home.

CHAPTER 10

Bill the Person

He was a principled man, deeply rooted in his Christian faith. His actions were governed by his ever consciousness of his Christian duty to do things the way God would want him to do things. He took disappointments in stride. There was never a "why me?" He learned to also be firm when he had to be. He developed the firmness after he saw that not all people do what is right.

My baby, about as good as any man will ever be!

The morning he was born, the doctor told me he had a little trouble getting him breathing, but other than that, everything was fine. He was a healthy baby and had a good disposition from the start. I was happy about his birth, but some people thought it a problem that I was soon to retire from the air force with a baby to raise. Some people after being in the military services so long were really afraid to retire. I was confident of my ability to transition to civilian life and live well. Little did I know the joy of having Bill would bring me.

He began going to preschool at the age of three. He was loved by everyone, and by then it was evident the he had that wonderful personality that won everyone's admiration.

After we moved back to Arkansas in 1977, Bill transitioned well, and later told me he marveled at how I managed to arrange Christmas for him while living in a trailer while having a house built.

The house was out in the country, and he loved that. He had a thing for all things military, and he loved to go out in the woods and play soldier. He rode a school bus to Dover, and he loved the school and most of his teachers. Needless to say, it was no surprise, by that time, that he was loved by all.

When he was eight, I saw his head moving from side to side as he sat up in bed, and I was so upset wondering what it could be, not something threatening the life of my baby, I hoped. We were lucky as it was a rolandic seizure, a childhood disorder that could be treated with Dilantin. He was on Dilantin for about two years, which took care of the problem.

Three-heelers were the thing out in the country; everybody had one, it seemed. I bought Bill a used one when he was about ten years old and was very strict about how he rode it, making sure that he understood how dangerous they could be if not handled properly. He had a tendency to be a daredevil from an early age, but he listened well and really enjoyed it without adding too many gray hairs for me. I sold the first one and bought him a new one in the fall of 1986.

His mother and I had never gotten along, and when we divorced in 1986, he stayed with me, with her concurrence. I had been fighting a back problem for years, but I hired someone to clean the house and he and friends mowed the grass and he and I had a wonderful life together. I would get him up, fix his breakfast, make his lunch and send him off to school, and have a meal for us each night. I don't remember the occasion, but he presented me an apron, which I still have and will always treasure.

We had three dogs, two outside and one inside. Buster, who looked a lot like a pit bull, was a very unusual dog. Bill had acquired him while we were in Florida. Butch, a German shepherd who had been acquired my son Steven in Florida, was the guardian of our ten acres; and Tippy ruled the inside of our home. Tippy, a poodle-Chihuahua mix, was bought to me while visiting a neighbor in Florida by Bill, and I told Bill that in no uncertain terms were we not going to keep him and for Bill to take him home. When I got home, there was Tippy, and Bill reminded me I had told him to take him home and he had. Shortly after we got him Tippy, he got distemper and had seizures and was sick for the rest of his life. Bill was jealous of the time and attention Tippy got, but I told him he must remember that Tippy was sick and I had to take care of him. Tippy died in 1988.

Bill would send me cards from him and the dogs after the divorce. Cards I still have and will always treasure.

We were very close, and I kept up with all his activities and whom he was with and in a case or two forbid his seeing certain kids. If he was out at night, I would not go to sleep until he came home. I made an exception to how late he could stay out on New Year's nights and he would call me at midnight and I would talk to him and Tammy Zachery and several of his friends and tell him to come home soon.

My baby, as I have referred and still refer to him as, had it at an early age; how could anyone not love him? Someone at his funeral said he lit up every room he ever walked in to.

My uncle Burford lived in Little Rock and was as bitter as his father had been. He so hated this country that after the September 11, 2001, terrorist attack he was so furious that so many people were flying the American flag. In spite of his hatred, he was always really impressed that my Bill was such an intelligent and good person.

Chapter 11

Conclusion

Bill always told me I didn't pay enough attention to many things, and he was correct. For some strange reason, I was a better observer than many people were when I was working.

Tom Peters, the management guru, used to write about many things, and one I picked up on was management by walking around. I've told some of my friends that I can walk into a business and see four or five things that I would change immediately. I guess some of it comes from being put in charge of functions that had not been managed well. I think mostly it's God given; just observe and pay attention when it is important to do so.

While I had jobs that called for people of a higher rank, I was a peon. I learned though, from studying the thinking and actions of more educated and higher-ranking people, that it is much better to look ahead and prevent problems than to solve them. I was always observing and thinking where things could go wrong and prevented many of the "unforeseen" things from happening. I think that is why I was successful where others had failed.

One thing I emphasized to Bill was sensible decision making. I told him many people fail because they do not analyze things sufficiently before making decisions. I recently noticed that Harvard has a home study course on decision making.

Bill proved that he had a good handle on it.

When I first read about management by walking around, I thought back and thought, well, I guess God was helping me when I needed it most. I would take over some function and observe a little while and call a meeting and make some changes.

I look back with real pride in that senior military officers and civilians placed so much trust in me.

The point I'm trying to make is to use your God-given abilities well.

I saw when Bill was young his abilities and knew he was to go far in this world, and he would have had not diabetes taken his life so young. I wanted him well educated so, as I told him, he would get well paid for his accomplishments and not make other people look good and not profit from his good decisions like I did many times.

He had no banking experience, but he talked about his and Jim's conversations so much that I knew Jim could see in him what I had seen in his early life. He said he had heard Jim was very upset over the problem he had been hired to clean up. When he told me about his and Jim's conversations, I knew Jim could see his real potential.

At the end of his workday at Arvest, he would go home and assist the kids with their homework and then start writing poems, screenplays, or whatever he was working on and he got very little sleep. I was very impressed at the visitation at the funeral home in Mountain Home, that there were so many little Cub Scouts circling his casket; I thought, that's my baby; he found time for the scouts also.

It took Lisa and me a long time to get to where we could live with his death better. On January 7 of 2009, she called me late in the day after work and asked me if I had been to his grave, crying. I told her no; I just had to go to his grave on Christmas Day. He always wanted me with him on Christmas Day, and his grave was as close as I could get to him. I met her and the kids in Conway and we talked and ate, and discussed how he might feel about how we have handled things after his death.

On January 7 of this year, 2010, I handled his death much better, and I think she did also. This was the fifth year after his death.

He truly was a special person. He never saw himself as having exceptional abilities, like others did. One of his grammar school teachers, Mrs. Griffith, said he talked too much in class, and I told her to whip him. She said, "Whip Bill!" and I said yes, and she looked at me like at me like I was a nut. Everyone loved him!

He was a fun-loving daredevil. But when it came to family, country, concern for others and his country, he always came down on the "do what is right" side. He never could understand how anyone could not believe in God. He would cite the miraculous things we see, the intricate workings of the human body, and other things that I believe most thinking people don't think just accidentally happened.

He was so cute in his '70s polyester coat and tie when he started preschool. His expression was kind of like "I'm the top dog around here," and he was loved by all.

We were close from the start. I guess I was too young to spend much time with my first two boys, but with Bill, it was like it didn't get any better than having a son like this.

When his mother and I got a divorce, we got along so well and I did things with him that I never did with my older boys. I was fighting a back problem, but when I could, we would go to stores that I had no interest in, like military surplus stores, and let him show me things, and I really enjoyed him. One day when he was a teenager, I was about to go in to Walmart and thought he would stay in our truck, but he insisted on going in with me. I said, "Not looking like that," and he gave me his impish look and insisted on going with me. Once inside, he paraded around like royalty, in his poorly dressed state. When we got back to the truck, I told him if he ever did that to me again, I would kill him. He was wearing a cowboy hat, combat boots, and shorts. I think he was kind of thinking like Drew; irritate Dad a little bit.

His kindness and consideration of others were natural from an early age. Shortly after he started driving, he came home one day and told me he had dodged a bird and had damaged the truck's front bumper a little. At first I was a little irritated but later thought, How can you be upset knowing he has a heart like that? I often called him my baby, and believe me, he was. I have to quit for a little while now!

Some understanding of my family life and how it affected Bill and me needs to be understood.

I met Bill's mother while stationed at Fort Chaffee, near Fort Smith, where she lived.

Her family was poorer than mine had been. Her mother was the boss at home, and her father, George, did what he was told to do. She tried to boss me around and tell me what to do at home and at work. She never under understood; I wasn't George. I knew what to do. I have never seen anyone who could spend so much money and never have anything to show for it.

After my back got so bad that I could no longer work, I had no choice but to get a divorce so I could control the reduced income I received and have enough for Bill and me to live. I was surprised that we managed to live so well, and I could then begin to invest a little.

Bill's brothers always listened to their mother, and I was always a nut as far as they were concerned. On the other hand, Bill adjusted to life as it is, early in his life. I remember telling a lady whose family had been very successful that my Bill had a better grasp of real life than most forty-year-olds did when he was still a teenager.

Looking back, it was good that I had to start helping my dad at an early age, as I learned how important it was to stretch every cent and make money go as far as possible and to think everything through before making decisions.

The fact that my other two sons would never listen to me is one of my greatest disappointments in life. I finally just cut off any further financial assistance when they were in their fifties. It was an easy decision as they had no respect for me.

Steven had now turned his life around, he has a wife who works and exerts spending controls, and they are doing well.

The fact that I had several very intelligent and successful friends only impressed my Bill, not my first two sons. He would remind me of that when I expressed my displeasure at never getting a college degree.

Bill always listened to me and didn't agree with his brothers' opinion of me, and he attributed his success in life to my guidance. He said I kept him from jumping into things without proper thoughts about things. When he was born, I told his mother that he wasn't going to be raised the way his brothers were. He listened to me, and when he heard how stupid his dad was, he didn't accept it.

When he wanted to become a JAG officer, I was really against it, but he loved our country and the military services and wanted to do his part to contribute to the defense needs of our great country. Diabetes had destroyed his chances to be either a commercial or military pilot, which he really wanted to do. He said the doctor who gave him his physical examination for JAG duty said they did not ask if he was a diabetic, so he approved his medical qualification.

He was commissioned as a first lieutenant and promoted to the rank of captain in about a year. Had he lived, about now he would have eligible for promotion to the rank of major.

Bill Self told me, soon after his death, that Ben would be just like his dad; and I didn't see it at the time, but now I do. When Ben was in the fourth grade, he was reading at the tenth-grade level, which shocked me at the time, but now I see that he is going to be as intelligent as his dad was. While I don't speak perfectly, I always tried to speak well. Ben is eleven now and recently, he, his mother, and sister, and I had a long conversation, and speaking well came up. I commented on how discouraged and displeased I was to hear so many people say "I seen." Ben told about several things he had heard, and I was so proud that he was so conscious that he at eleven noticed and was bothered by such poor speech.

When he was young, Drew was amazed at how I kept up with was going on in the world. Today he does the same thing. Bill did also.

Drew and his wife Jeanette and daughter Bailey own an Apple Spice Junction food catering business here in Little Rock. Jeanette is an RN who quit nursing to help Drew in the business. His family and I are close. If I need something, they expect me to call them, and that really means a lot. We hug when we meet and depart, just like Bill and I did. In fact, he and his family make sure that I am not alone on holidays, and they invite me to their home. I tell people that he is like another son, and he really is. Jeanette cried for nearly three years every time Bill was mentioned after his death.

Drew lost his dad, Joe, before we lost Bill. I didn't plan it (I wasn't capable of planning anything at that time), but Bill is buried beside Joe. Lisa's sister suggested that area of the cemetery for Bill. After we selected the two spaces, I looked to my right and saw Joe's grave and asked which space was Bill's and realized he was being buried by Joe. The question, how did that happen, will always linger.

I feel really more cared about by them than by my other two sons.

I lost my baby, but I have a wonderful daughter-in-law, who teaches kindergarten, and two wonderful grandchildren who are the joy of my life now. I tell Lisa often how lucky I am to have her raising my grandchildren. She told me that I just didn't realize how much he loved me. I told her I do, because I loved him the same way.

Bill and I had a broad range of interests, and we discussed practically everything that went on in the world. When I learned he had died, the first thing that came to my mind was that my baby and I could never talk again.

Much later that night, I couldn't sleep so I got up and drove for quite some time as I often did when I was troubled about something. I slept very little for about five or six days until I took some sleeping medication, which only helped some.

One of my fondest memories is him telling me that we loved each other as father and son and we were best friends. We really were; we could just do anything, simple things, and be together and enjoy it. If he felt like chewing me out, it was OK. I told one of his brothers that he had earned the right to do it. After he went to work as a lawyer and until he died, if he wanted to talk in the middle the night, he called and we talked. I told Lisa he never said "Dad, I need your opinion"; he just started talking about what troubled him, and I would hear him out, ask the questions I thought necessary, and then tell him how I would handle the situation.

He was so intelligent that I never understood his reasoning behind telling me that he would never have gotten to where he was had it not been for my advice.

If he had been able to go to the naval academy, his desire was to fly fighter aircraft. That not being possible, he thought of being a commercial pilot. Diabetes changed everything. He told me that having to give up flying was the hardest thing he had to learn to live with.

Once he adjusted to the realities of life, he would have been happy to pursue a business career. After he had cleaned up the situation he had been hired to do, he said he was willing to just clean up problems for Arvest for a few years and then settle down somewhere. He was waiting for Arvest to choose his next assignment when he died.

He had a total of about fifteen years of military service. After his active duty service, and prior to becoming a JAG officer, he had served as an enlisted man in the national guard and the reserves for several years. His view was that being a JAG officer allowed him to keep his ties to armed forces, which he loved so much.

My goal for him was that he become the chief executive officer of a billion-dollar company, and he was on his way. When I would tell him I was nowhere near him in education, he would say, "Dad, look who your friends are." He would say, "Dad, you came from nothing," and I would tell him that we should all just do the right thing and deal with hardships as they came and always strive to do what we knew was right and believe me, he practiced that all of short life.

When he was young, he would say things like "I don't got" and there was something else he said that I just, so far, cannot remember, which stood out because of his intelligence.

As I mentioned before, my dad stressed honesty in our lives. Bill would have been so loved by my dad as he lived a life of total responsibility for his actions and needs. When I offered to help him with his school loans, he said I had done enough by buying him two trucks. When he was buying a house in Mountain Home, he called me to deposit a thousand dollars in his checking account temporarily. A week or so later, he sent me a check for one thousand and ten dollars.

After his death I learned about so many things he had told about his and my life. I was surprised at how much the people whom he worked with knew about our lives. Bill Self said he talked about me all the time. We both loved to talk.

Bill was very jealous of my Yorkie Liz, but having her has helped me make the transition to life without him easier.

Folks, when you lose a child, it is never easy; losing one with a heart that was there for everything that lived and breathed was very hard to deal with.

It took about four and a half years for me to have a real interest to do anything I really wanted to do. Now, five years after he died, I have an interest in wanting to do things I enjoy again, like playing bridge and doing something I might enjoy. It has taken this long to accept that what has happened, happened, and yes, I am going to have to live without him. I have no other choice. But I will always know that I had one of the most honest, decent, principled men that God ever put on this earth.

He was so exceptional that I am sure God only made a few Bills.

God, thank you for giving me such a wonderful son!

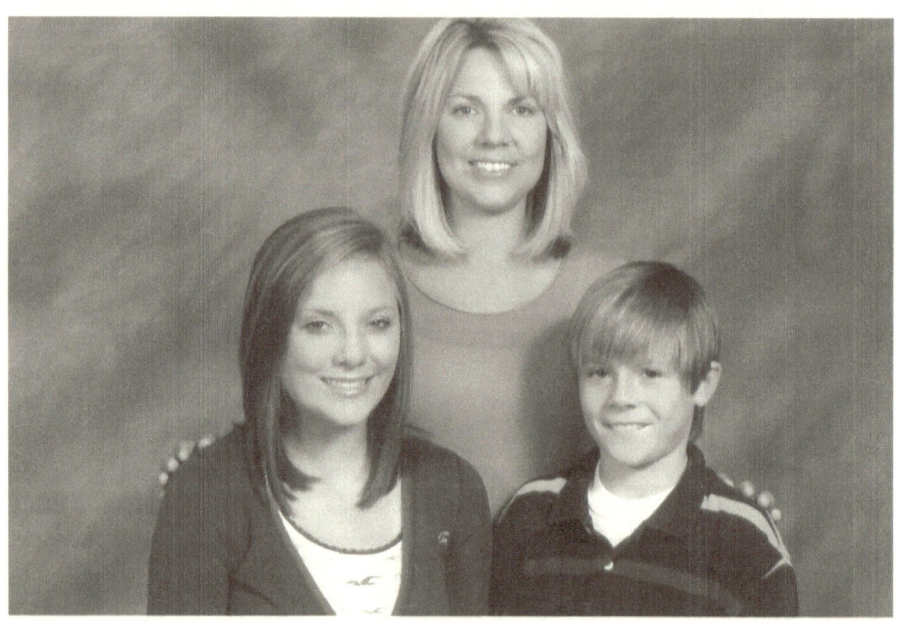

Lisa, Alexa and Ben

EPILOGUE

by Lisa

What do you say about a man whose funeral lasted two and one half hours? I mean, do you hear of that happening often? I never had before. Well, maybe in the movies, or for very famous people, but never "regular" people. My Bill was one of those rare, extraordinary, "regular" people. I say *my* Bill. I did not own him; he was not property, but he was *mine*. I had him for a wonderful thirteen years. He was mine and I was his. Saying *Bill and Lisa* was as synonymous as saying salt and pepper. What was I going to do without myself? Could they just go ahead and bury me right along with him? Maybe these thoughts ran through my mind as I sat there in a catatonic state at his burial, or maybe it was in the days before or after. Some of it is a blur now, but at some point the thought did occur to me. I wanted to go with him.

What a funeral it was. I suppose you would find it odd to hear someone say they didn't want a funeral to end, but I didn't want Bill's to end. It was filled with loving remembrances of him, funny stories I wanted to remember and hold on to, and tales of noble acts of character and Christianity that I wanted my children to hear. Most of all, the ending of the funeral meant he was really going to be gone. There in the church, he was lying in a casket in front of me, not breathing, but he wasn't *gone*. I could still see him. This could still be just a dream. There was still time for it to be a mistake. When he was put in the ground, there would be no more time. That cold, lifeless ground.

It was a bearable temperature for a January day. No rain. Turning into the cemetery, I looked back once. The funeral procession seemed to stretch for five miles. That's no surprise. Bill was so loved and admired. Anyone who ever met him had an immediate feeling that he was one of their closest friends. He was handsome, charismatic, smart, and funny. He made me laugh. He made everyone laugh. He was the headlining source of entertainment at social gatherings. In fact I think his burial was his final performance. As you read in the book, he had the honor of being given a military funeral, which includes a twenty-one gun salute. The first seven shots were fired, then silence, then the last seven shots fired. Every single soldier's rifle misfired on the second shot. Then coincidence? I don't think so.

Life without him has been hard. Not a single day has gone by that me and our children haven't thought of him and wish he were still alive with us. It has been painful to watch them suffer through milestones that should be shared with their dad. I see him in each of them. They got his "good stuff." But we are moving along every day, and I thank God that we had the blessing of sharing life with him even for a little while. I thank God that Bill is in the most wonderful place to be. I thank God that I will see him again someday. Everyone should enjoy the chance to have a Bill in their lives.

INDEX

A

Acxiom Corporation, 40–41
air bases
  Barksdale Air Force Base, 19
  Lowry Air Force Base, 21
  Selfridge Air Force Base, 23
  Tyndall Air Force Base, 22
  Wurtsmith Air Force Base, 24
Anderson, Allene (Mrs. Edwin Kurt Pusch),
    11, 26, 28
Anderson, L. D., 27
Anderson, Lula Bell, 11
Arvest Bank, 41, 43–45, 52, 55

B

Ben (Bill Pusch's son), 35, 42, 47, 54, 56
Blue Chip Ice, 34
Burford (Jack Pusch's uncle), 12–13, 27–28,
    36, 50
Buster (pet dog), 50
Butch (pet dog), 50

C

Church of Christ, 31, 35
Crumpler, Drew, 32–34, 53–54
Crumpler, Joe, 32–33, 54

D

Dame, Tom, 46
Dare, Frank, 31

E

Elmer (Allene's brother), 12–13

F

First Baptist Church, 35

G

Gerlach, John, 47
Griffith (grammar school teacher), 52
Grigsby, Scott, 46

H

Harwell, Lisa (Mrs. William Pusch Jr.), 34,
    36, 47, 52
Heatherington, Travis, 20
Hell's Half Acre, 11

J

James Benjamen (Bill Pusch's son). *See* Ben
Jeanette (Drew Crumpler's wife), 34, 54
Johnson, David, 47

L

Lee, Layton, 34
Lee, Robin, 34
Lewis, R. C., 48
Louise (Allene's sister), 13, 31

M

Mathews, Jack, 19
Matthews (lieutenant), 21
Mclemore, David, 35
Minton, Roy, 40, 52

N

94th Fighter Interceptor Squadron, 24

O

120th Medical Clearing Company, 17

P

Peters, Tom, 51
Pitman, Heather, 34
Pitman, J. J., 34
Pusch, Alexa, 34–35, 47
Pusch, Edwin Kurt, 19, 26
Pusch, Jack, Jr., 21–23, 29
Pusch, Jack, Sr., 24
   military career of, 16–25
   postmilitary career of, 29
   preteen years of, 11–14
   recollections of Bill by, 49–56

religious participation of, 31, 35
Retha Mae Winders's courtship with and
   marriage to, 53
return to Arkansas of, 30–31
teenage years of, 15
Pusch, Steven, Jr., 34
Pusch, Steven Kurt, 19, 21–23, 29, 34, 53
Pusch, William L. (Bill)
   acquisition of pilot's license by, 32
   death of, 46–47
   diagnosis of diabetes on, 35
   diagnosis of histoplasmosis on, 33
   education of, 32–34, 36
   funeral of, 47–48
   Lisa Harwell's courtship with and marriage
     to, 34–35
   military career of, 32
   professional career of
     with Acxiom, 40–41
     with Arvest, 43, 45–46
     with Rochelle, 38

R

Reidel, Amber, 34
Reidel, John, 34
Rochelle (law firm), 38–39

S

Sam (Jim Walton's father), 45
Second Baptist Church, 35, 47
Seitz, J. F. R., 18
Self, Bill, 47, 54–55
Self, Trieneke, 47
Shipley, Keith, 34
Stump, Carmen, 34
Stump, Heath, 34
Sydney (Dale Whitney's daughter), 38

T

Taylor, Frank A., 20–21
Thresher, Brad, 34, 41
Thresher, Melanie, 34
Tippy (pet dog), 50
Torrie (Dale Whitney's wife), 38

V

Vernon (Allene's brother), 13

W

Wainwright, Euel, 23–24
Walton, Jim, 44–46, 52
Whitney, Dale, 38
William (Allene's brother), 13
Winders, Retha Mae
        (Mrs. Jack Pusch Sr.), 16

Y

Young, Robert, 34
Young, Stephanie, 34

www.ingramcontent.com/pod-product-compliance
Lightning Source LLC
Chambersburg PA
CBHW020408290526
45785CB00005B/2472